My Rock and Roll Transplant Journey

John Hunt

CHAPTER ONE

I was told by a very good friend that this book should be called "The Heart of Rock and Roll Is Still Beating" but, I thought Huey Lewis might have an issue with that. And I like Huey too much to piss him off...

This chapter is to set the stage toward how I started my journey to a Heart Transplant.

I think I may have used each of my "nine lives".

Despite my always positive attitude, I have been at or close to death so many times. My mother always loved telling the story of how she was in labor for 23 hours and I was coming too early. She chose to marry a man who was not my father so "I would have a name" as my grandmother told her that she would have to abort me if she did not get married. Then, after she was taken to the emergency room at Leland Memorial Hospital in Riverdale, Maryland on a snowy winter night, the umbilical cord was wrapped around my neck as she continued to vomit. Each time she did, the cord continued to tighten around my neck and the doctors were forced to rush the delivery so I would not die before being born. I was born jaundiced at just four pounds and six ounces. This was the first of many "almost death" experiences that have made me as strong as I am today.

Through later research I learned I was entering this world as John, Paul, George and Ringo were taking the stage for the first time for a public concert in America, just three miles away in Washington, D.C. Maybe it was all the screaming fans, which history says could be heard for miles, that helped me come out into the light to this amazing journey called life.

My mother quickly divorced the man as he was in the military and he was transferred to the west coast. Two years later she married the man who she has always claimed was my "biological father". The two of them are still married today. They gave me five younger sisters but, never had another boy, despite many years of trying. Though, we never had much, we always had enough to get by. The house however was always stress filled as there was always doubt on who my "actual father" was, and my "dad's" mental issues. I always tried harder, with the thought that despite my good grades, advanced studies and hard work that I was never "good enough" This led to an enormous drive toward always trying to "be the best" but, ultimately may have led to my death...

The stress in my house continued until I found my true calling. In my freshman year at Chopticon High School we had a radio station called WCHS. I tried out and earned a position anchoring the Morning News and a lunchtime music show. The first words out of my mouth were, "Hi, I'm John Hunt and you're not", which I stole from Chevy

Chase on Saturday Night Live. I had found my true passion and one of my major causes of stress. By this point in my life I already was driven to be the best. I was already working toward becoming a perfectionist. No one would beat me up mentally more than myself. Not "the best I could be" but, wanted to do anything to rise to the top possible. A few months before my 16th birthday I got my first job at a local AM radio station, in Leonardtown, Maryland. The station had a very small signal range. It was 1000 watts during the day and just 500 watts at night. I worked the six to midnight shift Monday through Thursday. Even though my show only was able to be heard for about a 15 mile radius and my pay was minimum wage, which was just $3.25 an hour, I learned many aspects of radio as we wrote and read news, played music, entertained, took requests and actually interacted with listeners. The climb up the radio ladder became my only focus. That job was followed by a few small market gigs before making it to the Akron/Cleveland Ohio market at age 19. My radio career took me around the country to Atlanta and Savannah, Georgia, Houston, Texas, and to a small gold mining town named Elko, Nevada before ending up in Oregon. There are many other radio stories that are quite fun that I may have to save for a future book.

Now, working in radio in the 80's and 90's could have led to many addictions. I say this because after the doctors figured out that the main cause of my heart issues and later heart transplant was cardiomyopathy. The muscle surrounding the heart was completely eaten up and diseased. Often, this can be caused by use of cocaine. Now, I experimented with a few things, like weed and speed pills in my high school days. I'm not Bill Clinton, I did inhale. I had the occasional drink but, almost never to excess. Two major events lead to my fear of anything harder. First was the cocaine related death of a friend from my Bladensburg High School days, former Maryland Terrapin basketball star and number one draft pick of the Boston Celtics, Len Bias. To this day, I truly believe that he did not try cocaine before that day and it ultimately killed him on the spot. I also hope that many others learned from that dreadful day. Then, I have always loved the comedy of the late Robin Williams. In one of his early stand-up routines he said that "Cocaine was God's way of saying you're making too fucking much money".

As a fulltime radio host and Program Director, there were many opportunities for addiction. One time I walked into the studio where a record company rep had put a line of coke on the table next to my mixing board and made the offer that it was mine if, I played his artist's record. I lost my temper and threw him out of my studio saying, that, "If the record was any good, I'd play it. Otherwise, go screw yourself!"
I did have a weakness that, as time went on caused large amounts of stress and took a few pieces of my old heart on the way. Women. So many beautiful women. With my constant need to be "good enough" I felt the need to be

with as many women as often as possible. Plus, Eddie Murphy said in his stand up, "even ugly guys can get 'lovin', look at Mick Jagger. (I always thought about guys like Tom Petty, Billy Joel and Bob Dylan, super talented, not pretty boys) I was never the hottest guy in the room but, was slightly funny and always tried harder. This was also just before the days when "safe sex" was talked about on a regular basis. Between the age of 15 and 30 well, let's just say the "number" was higher than I could count. I am lucky to have only two children because of my lack of restraint during this time. During the pre-transplant testing, where they test you for EVERY possible disease, especially the social diseases, I was so relieved that I did not have any of them. Every blood test came back completely clean. Of the 37 tests they gave me, that was the only one that scared me even in the slightest.

At age 24 I met and immediately fell in love with Kerry Elizabeth, the most amazing goddess I had ever met. We married and it was like living in a fantasy world. Everything was so perfect. Sure, we were young and had financial struggles but, no one had ever completely loved me and would have done anything for me like she did. But, after working in various nightclubs, spinning the turntables for a few years, and women offering anything I wanted up every night, I broke down and cheated. This mistake on my part caused my heart more stress than I had ever known and has haunted me ever since in one way or another. The crazy thing is, Kerry begged for me to stay in the relationship and fix the problems. I tried to be noble and told her that "I did not deserve someone as amazing as her" and gave up. In the entire relationship she only did one thing that could have been considered as a mistake or a lack of judgement and I made more than my share of bad judgements. We never argued or fought and there was never any abuse of any kind except for my one-time infidelity. I later learned that we could have fixed things even after my children were born. I was too stubborn to go back and paid a pretty heavy price. The next relationship led me to heart attack number one at age 35.

The final straw that led to me leaving the perfect relationship is when the woman I cheated with told me that she was pregnant. I had been telling friends that I was going to end things with her and fix things with my wife and she got wind of this. She cooked up a plan to keep me by telling me that she was with child. I then tried to "do the right thing" and be a good father. Two months later she claimed she had "lost the baby". I felt bad and did not leave at that time and a few months later she did get pregnant with the first of two amazing children. Even though I was not in love with her, I was in love with my son. I tried to stay in the relationship but, we realized a few years later that we were not in love and began packing things to go our separate ways. My father had a heart attack and had been given his first stent. He and my mother stopped by our townhouse on his way home after his hospital release when she announced to my parents, before I even knew, that she was pregnant again. I agreed a second time to stay in the relationship "for the sake of the kids". After my daughter was born, we had an on again, off again relationship for a while, and after a few years, she admitted that she was never pregnant the first time and that "God had spoken to her in an audible voice and told her to come clean with the truth.' Essentially this revelation completely ended the relationship.

CHAPTER TWO

Both of my parents have some sort of heart issues. However, none of my sisters have any known heart disease. My father has had two mild heart attacks that led to him having stents inserted to keep arteries open. My mother has dealt with an irregular heartbeat and heart murmur since she was in her twenties. They are both still alive into their middle 70's.

My first heart attack came at age 35. I was in the best physical shape of my life and was in perfect health. Or so I thought. I was working out regularly and was taking a pill that I got from GNC that made my body not hurt after a hard workout as building muscle comes from tearing and healing of the muscle. I was completely toned and had no intent on becoming Arnold Schwarzenegger or Charles Atlas, just wanted to be able to see the tone.

I was taking Androstenedione mixed into a vitamin pill before each workout. This is the same natural steroid that was found in Mark McGuire's locker that started the whole steroid controversy in Major League Baseball. I was under a ton of stress in my personal and work life and with my children's mother. My daughter Casey had been sick with a severe cold for a few days and did not want to be held by anyone but me. At the time she was only 2 years old. Whenever I tried to lay her down or give her to her mother she cried. So, I held her basically for three consecutive days, she would only sleep in my arms. I was extremely tired and as she began to improve, her mom started to argue loudly with me again and again. At this point I began to have severe chest pains. She did not believe I was being serious, and this led to a more heated argument. After I convinced her that this was serious, I went to Piedmont Hospital in Atlanta, Georgia. The doctors and ER staff did not believe I was having a heart attack saying that I was "so young and in such great shape". The pain started to subside only after they gave me Nitroglycerine tablets and they decided to keep me overnight for a stress test first thing in the morning.

I remember the Cardiologist saying, "I'm not sure why you are here. I'm sure you don't have any heart issues. You look way too good". When I started running on the treadmill my chest started hurting almost immediately. Then they did the old-fashioned test where they shoot isotopes into your blood and put me on the rotating MRI machine. The images showed "Something dark" in the photos and they decided to do my first catherization. Before my transplant, I had a total of 12 different heart catherizations. Some through the vein in my groin, some through my wrist and upper arm. The next morning, they sent me into an extremely cold operating room naked with only a small towel covering my shriveled privates. Yes, "shrinkage" in the cold is a real thing for guys! After going up through my thigh with the scope, the doctor then said to me, "I'm sorry Mr. Hunt but, you have a 99 percent blockage here." They proceeded to give me the first of nine stents that were in my old heart before the transplant. My recovery went very quickly, and I was back to work and coaching my pee wee hockey team on their opening game within two days. The doctors instructed me to take a basic statin to prevent blood clots and baby aspirin. I then took another stress test one year later and passed it with flying colors. I was taken off the baby aspirin and the statin at that time. At this point, I thought I was home free from any heart issues. I did not have any regular checkups and went another seventeen years before I had any additional heart problems.

During those years I ate healthier than I previously had, tried to stay in shape and had only a few health issues. Starting in 2009, I was working long days and met Katrina, a stunning woman who was amazing. She had just come out of a bad marriage and we had a great relationship. I went back to feeling like I was not good enough for this Wiccan Goddess and kept myself under constant stress as I went through battles in business as I fought to start a new enterprise in my radio career. In 2013 I was working long days and started to have severe pain in my abdomen. I tried to fight through it not wanting to miss any work. After about twelve days of this intense pain, I finally checked myself into Civista Hospital in LaPlata, Maryland. I then learned that again, I was lucky to be alive as I had a burst appendix that has the poison spread all throughout my stomach. They couldn't operate as they were afraid that poison might get into my blood stream if they did. I had a tube coming out of my stomach for over three weeks as they slowly drained the poison from my system, hoping it would not get into my blood. After my full recovery, I went back to work immediately. Also, at this time, everyone in the house was unable to do much as they were all either sick, injured or way too busy. So, as I noticed that the grass was way too high on our yard, and on a sunny, humid 95-degree Maryland day, I decided to cut the grass with a push mower. The lot was about 2 acres and I got about 90 percent of it done before coming in the house and collapsing. I woke up shortly afterward and realize that I was in major pain.

I was having trouble breathing and felt extremely dizzy and weak. I rested and never went to the doctor. I had issues for a few days but, recovered fully. Later, the doctors said that was either another heart attack or maybe a mild stroke.

I loved Katrina and her family dearly but, started to realize that my ultimate dream had always been to own my own radio station. That opportunity was on the West Coast and after some major discussions, we agreed that I would chase that dream and hopefully she would follow later or, I would be able to do a bunch of travel back and forth with all the money I believed I would make as an owner. I initially moved to Elko, Nevada as an owner that I had worked for previously was hoping to sell a few of his stations. We had our disagreements in the past but, he badly needed a good radio talent and sales guy and, I desperately wanted to be an owner. After I realized that I was being taken advantage of, and that deal may never be able to actually happen, my broker called me to tell me that I should not buy those underperforming radio stations and he had the perfect deal in a beautiful small town on the south coast of Oregon. I visited the town and immediately knew that this was the perfect deal. In Coos Bay, Oregon. A small coastal town about 90 minutes west of Eugene and 3 hours south of Portland.

The dream was becoming real...

CHAPTER THREE

My visit to Coos Bay and the decision to purchase the station came during a time in August 2015 when I was given the perfect "Chamber of Commerce" weather. Light breezes 75 degrees and sunshine every day. Even though I had done my homework and read that Oregon is one of the rainiest places in the USA, I decided to make the move. I left Elko in October 2015 and started my new life building my own station. It was the beginning of a dream come true.

At this point Matthew was finding his way as a video genius in Washington, DC and Casey was close to graduating with honors from Penn State University. Life was good. I was in love with a great woman and I was finally realizing my lifetime dream at age 51. I was beginning to feel that all the bad karma for mistakes I had made at a much younger age was gone. My attitude was positive but, I had much to learn about life on the west coast. On the east coast, I was always taught to go, go, go, don't stop until the project is done, dominate and be the best. I had so many struggles when I first arrived as I had to learn that the pace was not the same here. I was pushing myself way too hard. I should have known that 18-hour days and a family history of heart disease wouldn't mix

I spent the first few months setting things up as I was waiting for the FCC to approve the sale of the station to me. I found a new location, building and painting the new studio and offices, started meeting clients and setting up some big events. On Christmas Eve 2015 I was given an awesome present as the FCC called with my license approval. I scraped together everything I had financially and got a small loan and signed the deal to make KYSJ, The Wave 105.9 FM mine. We went "live" for the first time February 3, 2016 and even before I had a staff, I tried to break the Guinness Book Of World Records time for longest amount of consecutive time on air live. The record was just over nine days. The rules allowed for five minutes of time per hour off air. I would bank those hours so I could sleep at my apartment that was less than a mile away for just 90 minutes a night, then a quick shower and back to the studio. People delivered food to me to help my quest. I pushed myself to seven days and 9 hours before complete exhaustion set in. Then after just one day of rest, I began to bring in my staff that included a midday talent named Lexi and an afternoon guy named Travis. The area had not seen or heard anything like what we were doing for many years as we were completely live and local. Announcers in the studio from 5:30am when I arrived until 10pm when Travis left. We played "The Most Eclectic Mix of All That Rocks" rather than the same twenty songs over and over, like the other stations did. Then we set up the first ever South Coast Music Awards at the Egyptian Theatre, an antique theatre that held just over 300 people to honor as many of the local musicians as I could. It was a big production and was lucky enough to have the finest musicians in town play with other musician in other bands in a full Grammy Awards style. It was a "dress to impress" event and even though there was a ton of stress leading up to the event, we pulled it off without any major issues. I had a great stage manager and a team of announcers that helped the event run smoothly. I was beginning to get tired but, was having so much fun building my dream I couldn't stop. My day started at 4:30 every day and would not end until after 10 pm. I lived on four hours of sleep a night, seven days a week. Then I set up and paid for, our first in what we planned to be many bigger concerts. Things were going perfectly, and the community was getting excited to have The Reverend Horton Heat, a rockabilly band with radio airplay and a few hits come to town. A few days before the event, I had gotten word that at least one of my employees was skimming money and giving away tickets but, I did not believe it. I defended them constantly but, the stress was building. Then it happened...

Two nights before the concert I was unable to get to sleep. My heart was racing and then I would get a high fever and the room was spinning. I started to have serious chest pain, my shoulders hurt, and my left arm was numb. Here we go, all the signs they tell you about. I tried to get myself through it but, the issues continued. I then got in my car and drove myself to Bay Area Hospital which was just about two miles from my house. I stumbled in and the doctors immediately started working on me. I was in and out of consciousness and kept hearing them say "this guy needs to go to Eugene; we aren't able to do this here". I hardly knew anyone in Coos Bay and knew no one in Eugene. I remember begging them to "get it done here" and the next thing I knew I was on the operating table. They went in, cleaned out the two blockages and put in two stents. After I woke up, I realized that I needed to be out of the hospital so we could get the concert planning done. The doctors were not going to let me out and I almost pulled out the IV's as there were numerous problems happening with the concert and the band almost pulled out a few times. I was getting non-stop phone calls in the hospital with people telling me all the. work we had done was falling apart due to the inability to get anything done at the venue. Then Travis, with some help, took charge of the situation and even though the concert started late, it finally happened. I got many comments from listeners happy that we had made such a big act available to them in such a small town. Unfortunately, I had missed it.

After getting out of the hospital and counting the money and tickets, I realized that the rumors were correct and I learned that two, possibly three employees skimmed from the profits by giving away tickets to friends or pocketing the money. One of them admitted what he had done and repaid the funds. It was at this point I realized that this would be harder than I ever expected. I then felt the need to do almost everything myself as my trust was failing with most of my employees. Not only were my salespeople not working hard but, now they were stealing from me. This was not a big corporation; it was just me and my little LLC.

Shortly after this I had a planned trip back to the east coast to see Casey graduate from Penn State and was excited to see my lady goddess again. The graduation went well, but it was at this point that my heart was broken in a different way. The woman I hoped to build a future for then told me that she couldn't be in our relationship anymore after six years together. Even though I understand why she did not want to move west, I was crushed and then buried myself into my work even more. Nothing was going to stop me now. I was going back to the west coast do prove to everyone that I could make this a successful radio station and maybe I would even win her back.

My stress levels had shot to new highs as I immediately faced battles on the street in sales as the competition was constantly attacking my station. One unscrupulous rival salesman had the balls to say I was going to "throw in the towel and move back east" after my heart attack. Really? This guy obviously did not know who he was dealing with so, I began to go on the attack. The station on air was dominant and we did things that made the listeners unable to change the dial. I had a great air team who dominated the airwaves, we constantly had businesses and bands in the studio live, which entertained the listeners. On the financial end, it was a constant struggle to make progress as it was hard to find many salespeople who wanted to dig in and work. Plus, there were our share of internal station battles to deal with amongst my sales team. There are many stories there which I will save for the "radio book".

Due to my insane work style, I was losing weight and getting sicker and more tired. It started with getting colds, and then in November 2016 I got a severe case of Influenza A. The doctors at Bay Area Hospital treated and released me with medicine to fight the flu. I kept working to work every day and collapsing at night. Then I started gaining weight extremely quickly. I was in and out of the hospital 12 times with the flu and the doctors would keep me overnight, drain me of fluids and send me home. I would feel better for a few days and would get back to work again immediately. I could barely walk up and down the steps from my studio to my office. My normal weight was about 175-180 pounds but, my weight kept ballooning to 215-225 pounds. The doctors gave me Torsemide to help me drain fluids more but, nothing was working. I had been working for a week on live broadcast remotes in Bandon, a beautiful beach town about 25 miles south of Coos Bay. After the last day of remotes, I was exhausted, I called Travis, and asked him to pick up the equipment as I was exhausted. I told him I was going home to sleep, and he yelled at me saying, "get back to the hospital, this has gone on too long, you have to fix this before you kill yourself!" I drove to Bay area Hospital for visit number 13. He met me there with his girlfriend and the ER techs found my blood pressure to be 59 over 40. The techs kept bringing other blood pressure machines to see if that one was broken but, the first one was accurate. They kept asking how I was even talking and joking with them. I was then checked into a room, ordered dinner and then started the wildest journey of my life...

CHAPTER FOUR

Am I Dead Now?

Many have said there is a "bright white light" when you see the other side. Others say, you are in total peace and find a new consciousness. I am not sure, but I get asked on a regular basis, "What Is it like being dead" or What did you see on the other side". When I woke up from falling asleep in Coos Bay, I learned that I had been in a coma for six days after I died twice in Coos Bay and revived both times. I awoke in the Intensive Care Unit at Oregon Health and Sciences University Hospital in Portland, Oregon. As I was waking up, the first thing I remember were the smiling faces of Dr. Jonathan Davis and Dr. Divya Soman (who was a Fellow at the time). The first words I remember were Dr. Davis saying, "Welcome back Mr. Hunt, we weren't sure if you would be joining us again. Your children are on a plane now from Washington, DC and think they are coming to say goodbye" The doctors said that I started to function one day earlier but, slipped back into the coma after just a few hours. I do not remember any of that. All that I can remember from those six days was having long but, choppy dreams. Just like in the movies, when a guy is about to be in a fatal crash and his life flashed before his eyes. I remember that the dreams were bits of memories of great things my children had done through the years like Matthew playing hockey and football, or Casey getting academic awards and cheerleading, trips we had taken together and the fun times I had interviewing people or doing my radio shows. I did not see the bright light or the fires of hell...I guess neither side was ready for me yet!

I had wires and tubes coming out of my neck and chest as well as my private parts like I had never seen before. As soon as I woke up., I wanted to get up and get back to work but, was told that I would be a visitor in the City of Portland for several weeks, possibly months. Matthew and Casey showed up a few hours later and were happily surprised to see me awake. To me, that was the greatest reunion of all time, as I had not seen them since Casey's graduation from college. The doctors let the kids and I know that I was about to start a long road to recovery. This was the first time that the words Heart Transplant were brought up as even a possibility. Dr. Davis explained that I may have been dealing with my cardiomyopathy for years, and the muscle around my heart was already about 80 percent dead. This left my heart unprotected and the flu I got in Coos Bay immediately attacked my unprotected heart.

It was then that I met Dr. James Mudd. I asked him where he was from and he told me Montana. I asked where he went to college and he said Johns Hopkins in Baltimore, Maryland. I told him that I knew a story about a famous Dr. Mudd from Maryland. Dr Mudd had a unique name to anyone from Maryland. As a child we went on History class field trips to the Dr. Mudd House in Bryantown, Maryland. Dr Samuel Mudd was the doctor who in 1864, set the leg of John Wilkes Booth, the assassin of President Abraham Lincoln. And because he was doing his job fixing Booth's leg as he was running from the police, Dr. Mudd was named a co-conspirator in the assassination of Lincoln. A charge he fought until his death. Dr. James Mudd was a direct descendant of Samuel Mudd. Proving that it truly is a small world.

Dr. Mudd told me that he would be putting a defibrillator and pacemaker into my chest to help keep me going as they mapped out a possible plan toward a Heart Transplant. They started a regiment of blood pressure meds, blood thinners and a diuretic to make things easier in my dying heart. I also was on IV heart pump meds they called "rocket fuel" also known as Dobutamine. It was used to "tune up" my heart and hopefully make it stronger so it could begin working on its own again. I also worked with Dr. Jill Gelow, the fourth member of the team and even though I did not see her much, she was an amazing cardiologist as well.

Through the whole process I made friends with many members of the team at OHSU from food service people (and the food was very tasty at this hospital, even though I was on a low sodium and heart healthy diet.) I felt especially bad one night, as the doctors were trying to lower the Dobutamine (They called it my "rocket fuel". Does that make me a "Rocket Man now?) and I got up to urinate. As I finished, I realized that I was getting weak and began throwing up everywhere just as my favorite nurse, Kimberly walked in. It was the biggest mess I had ever witnessed, and she graciously had it cleaned up as I felt horrible and profusely apologized. She along with many others there were top notch and I continually called OHSU the "Top Gun" of hospitals. The best of the best. I also remember a CNA named Danielle who always took the extra time to see how I was and told me stories about her latest dating escapades and ice cream dates. I also had an amazing view of the City of Portland and the south waterfront for six weeks after I was released from the ICU. This helped me start my love affair with Portland.

At this point my ejection fraction was between nine and twelve percent. A "normal" ejection fraction is anything over 55 percent. The ejection fraction is a measurement of the percentage of blood leaving the heart each time it contracts. The team at this point realized that a Heart Transplant was at some point inevitable. Not a question of "if" but, "when". The hope was to keep my own heart working, even at a slower pace for as long as possible and to do it with no "bridge to transplant" such as a heart pump. There was no need to do any type of bypass as the damage was too far along to fix the heart and the arteries. The doctors started the run of every imaginable blood test, gave me every booster shot for immunization, did tests like bone density and cat scans and even gave me the always fun, colonoscopy, which came out with no cancer or polyps, but, I started to wake up before they were finished and could see the TV showing the scope up my buttocks. It looked like that show "The Fantastic Voyage" where they travel through the human body. Good thing they cleaned everything out of there with the nasty tasting "lemon flavored" substance, that I had to drink two gallons of the night before surgery. The reason for all the tests is to be sure you are not going to die of something else and waste a perfectly good and very hard to come by, donor's heart. Then there are the psychological tests to be sure you won't jump off the top of a thirty-story building with the gift of someone else's heart. And the favorite of all is to be sure you have full and complete insurance coverage to the cover the multi-million-dollar cost of the Heart Transplant itself. Plus, the follow up work and medicines. It always made me think I was going to be like, "Steve Austin, astronaut. A man barely alive. Gentlemen, we can rebuild him..." (with the vision of a slow-motion running man...)" Better than he was before. Better, stronger, faster..." I had passed every test with flying colors. I was the perfect human specimen, except for the dying heart. Kind of like having a great car with an engine that doesn't make the car go.

During this time, I was chomping at the bit to get back to Coos Bay and the radio station. I was hearing the trash that was being talked about me "still being dead" and that I would never be healthy enough to broadcast again". I was also getting hundreds of calls each day with people taking the time to check on me and to show their support but, I was not ready to speak to anyone except for Lexi,

Travis and my family. So, I came up with a crazy idea to pass the time in my hospital bed and get some work done so I would not go completely crazy. I remembered a scene in a movie called "Pirate Radio" where Phillip Michael Hoffman, who was a DJ on the ship broadcasting illegal rock and roll back to England in the 60's said, "They can't stop us, we're pirates. I'll be broadcasting from this station until the day I die. And then probably a few days after that!" I called Travis and we figured out a way to have me record about 15 breaks each night and he would play them on air with the appropriate music to follow. It sounded like I was in the studio again. The doctors initially had their doubts about letting me do this but, I assured them this would help keep me sane during the long hospital visit. Word got around the hospital that I was doing this, and hospital administration paid me a visit saying they would cut off my room's internet if I continued as they were worried about possible HIPPA violations. I told them why I was doing the broadcasts and that the doctors had approved the broadcasts. She came back the next day and said that it would be acceptable if, I only talked about my health and things that went on in my room. A few of the doctors and other staff were listening to the broadcasts through our phone app. One of the members of the food service team delivered my food and told me had a cousin who was a big fan of The Wave and lived in Coos Bay and had heard me talking about how delicious the food was and how awesome the delivery people were. He always made sure after that that

I got some special combinations added to my choices, within my diet restrictions, of course.

The team at OHSU had done an amazing job at "Tuning me up" and making me as strong as I possibly could be. But there was still just one problem. As I was living in Oregon alone, I had no family or significant other in the State Of Oregon, I would not be able to get the transplant at OHSU and they said that I needed to go home to the east coast immediately. Do not pass go, do not collect $200.00.

It was time to go home...

CHAPTER FIVE

I ended up moving in with my son, Matthew and his two roommates in a one bedroom with a loft, apartment in Washington, DC and began my time at Washington Hospital Center. At which point I was told that "I did not meet the threshold for transplant" as OHSU had "tuned me up too well" Despite two overnight visits after having "mild" heart attacks, my status did not change with them for six months. During the time in D.C. I spent time rebuilding damaged relationships with one of my sisters, and my parents and strengthened a great relationship with another. I felt like I was driving everyone around me crazy, so, I decided to head back to Oregon where I knew I would be under better care in OHSU's heart program. Initially, I moved in with roommates and finalized the deal to sell the radio station. Selling the radio station was a sad day for me but, I realized that I was bleeding money trying to keep it going and found a deal that was very close to allowing me to break even financially and it drastically lowered my stress level. In February 2018, I moved to Portland permanently, and restarted the journey with OHSU to get me to transplant. I had a few friends that agreed to state that they would stay with me for the required three months after transplant and Matthew moved closer as he got a job in Los Angeles, California, which is just a short plane ride to Portland. This was enough to satisfy the team at OHSU. I then started cardio rehab and a drug study for the heart drug Entresto. My ejection fraction continued to drop, and I had three more heart attacks including one "Widowmaker" that completely blocked the arteries on the left side of my heart. I drove myself to each of those hospital stays as well. I was learning the difference between mild chest pain and a full heart attack.

The doctors on the team started to believe it was very close to time for me to get officially listed for transplant as I was sliding down the cliff very quickly. I was hanging on by my fingernails but, we all knew that it was very close to transplant time. Something was happening to cause the doctors to delay listing me for transplant but, I could not figure out what it was. Then, came one of the scariest days in my Heart Transplant journey. It was a day that I never saw coming and it was a shock to the entire OHSU Heart Transplant community. At this time there were nearly 350 patients waiting to be listed for transplant, 20 on the waitlist and another 327 in various phases of after transplant care. The program was the only Heart Transplant program in the State of Oregon and had, according to statistics from The National Registry of Transplant done anywhere from 15 to 27 transplants a year over the previous ten years. The data showed that OHSU had a demand that was higher than the national average, and 17 percent died in Oregon waiting for transplant compared to just eight percent nationally.

Then I went in for a follow up visit with Dr. Mudd, in October of 2018, and he dropped a bomb on me.

Dr Mudd was in tears as he explained that OHSU had decided to completely drop their Heart Transplant program. All other transplants would still happen there but, no more Heart Transplants. I also had meetings with Dr. Soman and Dr. Davis who were both visibly upset over their leaving OHSU. The administration was telling the patients initially that the program would be back to normal in "a few weeks" which later turned into "a few months" and then came the announcement that the program was ending "indefinitely". The real story, coming from the doctors stated that when they all were hired, they were told there would be six to eight doctors in the program and they all were working 60 to 80-hour weeks and were constantly on call. Dr. Gelow asked to have her hours cut back as she wanted to adopt a child. The administration denied her request, so she resigned and moved to Providence Hospital, where she is now my Portland Cardiologist after transplant. When the other three doctors asked if OHSU would be hiring more doctors they were told by the administration, that would not be happening. At this point, these very talented doctors all decided to resign and take their talents elsewhere. Dr Davis to The University of San Francisco, Dr. Mudd to Providence Hospital in Spokane, Washington and Dr. Soman to Kaiser Permanente in Clackamas, Oregon. With the program in shambles, each of us was off to find someone to get us to transplant. I transferred to Providence St Vincent's where Dr. Gelow set me up with Dr. Abraham and Dr. Westerdahl who kept me steady until we were able to start work at The University of Washington Hospital in Seattle. The doctors knew I need a transplant soon but, were not overly worried because my blood type is AB Positive. This blood type can be a blessing or a curse when it comes to transplants. An AB Positive can accept either an AB an A, B or O. However, an AB positive donor can ONLY go to another AB positive recipient.

In March 2019, while waiting for my transplant, Nike co-founder, Phil Knight and his wife Penny, decided to donate $75 million to Providence Health and Services to develop a new Heart Transplant program. Within 30 minutes of the Providence news conference, OHSU announced that it was rebuilding its heart program. Coincidence? I think not. Phil Knight had also donated millions of dollars to OHSU in previous years with most of it going toward the design of a fully artificial heart, a program that was also scrapped with their transplant program. Providence is expecting to begin transplanting hearts in March or April 2020 and OHSU has no known timetable for their first potential Heart Transplant.

Despite the delays and the fact that this journey from my death to possible transplant was nearing the two-year mark, I still believed that something amazing was going to happen, and soon.

CHAPTER SIX

From the moment I arrived at The University of
Washington hospital, things seemed different. I had gone
from someone that everyone knew, to just a number and
a chart. Or so I thought. I was greeted by my first
Transplant Coordinator, Sue Moore who was very direct,
professional and to the point. She knew that things
needed to progress quickly and how severe my condition
was, and she was amazing at making things happen. I
would be starting all the tests, except the colonoscopy
over again. The first was the blood draw where they took
27 vials of blood and they had me fill two cups on the
urinalysis. We redid the bone density and CAT scans,
breathing and oxygen tests. I had visits with a nutritionist,
infectious diseases and the psychologist. I met my Heart
Transplant Surgeon Dr. Koomalsingh and we joked that
like the TV commercial for AT&T where the doctor had
"just gotten back from suspension" that "Just OK was not

OK". Financial Planning and the Social Work departments jumped into action immediately as I was approaching the finish line to finally be listed for transplant. Within three weeks all the tests were completed and two years to the day that I had initially died in Coos Bay and went into the coma, I got the call that the doctors had all agreed that I would be listed for transplant at "Level 6". This was May 7, 2019. The rating system had recently changed so my pre-transplant coordinator explained that a Level One was in the hospital and near death. Two was on certain meds and about to enter the hospital, three was a patient in severe shape but, living at home, and so on. I was a SIX! This could take forever! Plus, I was an AB Positive blood type! Would I ever find the perfect heart match? I was told to "keep a bag packed but, the transplant might not happen for six months to a year as there were so many on their list due to the fact that many patients had been transferred to them after OHSU shut down it's transplant program. Before this, they were listed in many reports as in the top three in every report, showing that they did the most transplants and they were the most successful with a 91 percent success rate for transplant patients at least one year after their surgery. My brain and old heart were racing as I prepared to be patient and wait and always kept my sense of humor and positive attitude about the whole situation. Everything was happening for a reason; I just did not know what it was yet. Then it came...Another huge shock.

CHAPTER SEVEN

I was living my life day to day, afraid to think long term about anything. I wouldn't even buy tickets to a concert unless it was happening that week. I would not make plans for trips too long in advance. I had been living with Suzie for awhile and things were basically good between us. We had nothing going on physically as certain parts of my body did not work very well for me due to the blood thinners that I had been on. We enjoyed each other's company and did things together like Portland Trailblazers Basketball games and dinner dates. I had a ticket to see The Trailblazers playoff game six against Denver for a shot to make the Western Conference Finals against Golden State. Damien Lillard had already hit the shot that put the dagger in Oklahoma City ending their season with a 45-foot bomb as he waved goodbye to Russell Westbrook. The greatest shot I have ever seen in NBA history. Suzie's mom stopped by and the plan was for us to pick Suzie up from work and head to the game. I was fully dressed for the game with my red "Rip City" shirt and Blazers ball cap on. This night would be an exciting one! I had no idea HOW exciting until I got THE CALL.

It was just TWO DAYS after being listed and got a call on my phone from a strange 800 number. In this day of robocalls and scams, I almost did not answer. I noticed the call was coming from Ohio. The pre-transplant coordinator had told me the company that made the heart matches was called "Buckeye" and they were based in north western Ohio. I figured they might have some questions so, after a few rings I answered. The caller said that they had found the "perfect match for my heart" and I "needed to get to Seattle immediately". Initially, I thought this may be a joke. I do have friends that would see the humor so, at first I said, "OK well, it's 5:00 in Portland, traffic sucks and I'm heading to the Blazers playoff game. Can I head to Seattle after the game?" She proceeded to tell me that this was not a joke and that they had found the perfect AB Positive match. It was not a "high risk" heart and I would never find a better match. Hearts from donors that ate known as "high risk" are those who have been in prison, have infectious diseases, people who had an "alternative lifestyle" or even people who have tattoos. They had even just started to allow Hep C hearts to be used in transplants with the recipient's permission. If you accepted one of these, you had a higher chance of rejection or infection but, they could begin treating whatever the disease was as soon as you received the new heart. Buckeye assured me that I would NEVER find a better more perfect match and after I picked my jaw up from the floor, I agreed to go to Seattle immediately. I called Matthew, Casey and Suzie and told them the news. I drove to my own transplant alone as Suzie chose to go to the game. Matthew flew up from LA immediately and Casey stayed in DC as she was graduating from George Mason Law School the next day. I was supposed to fly out after the game to DC and watch the ceremony. I then went on Facebook Live to post a video explaining what was happening and that I realized that this could be my last post ever and I had accepted where I had been in life. I added that I was ready for wherever the next step took me. The immediate response was amazing from all my friends and the rest of my family. It was "Showtime"! I grabbed a few things and started the drive toward Seattle in heavy rush hour traffic. As this was a Friday night, I was having trouble reaching my coordinator to ask her a few questions. For example, was I allowed to eat anything? Where in the hospital would I go? About an hour into the drive an assistant called me and told me that I needed to eat immediately as it would be my last opportunity to eat for awhile and where to go to in the hospital. I immediately stopped in Kelso, Washington and ate at Red Lobster. A sweet waitress named Alexandra saw that I was all dressed in my Blazers outfit but seemed out of sorts. She asked "Is everything OK? What are you doing here? Isn't the game starting?" I then explained this was my "Last Supper" before a Heart Transplant. She was so nice with many questions about how I was handling everything. I paid my bill, and as I walked to my car another lady came running out to my car trying to get my attention. The General Manager of the restaurant asked me to come back inside as she had something for me. Alexandra had told her about the pending transplant, and she gave me $50.00 in gift certificates for "after I got better" and she wanted to be sure I came back to visit them again. It was a very touching gesture that took my mind off the journey in front of me for a few moments. Then back to the car to finish the trip. I was able to listen to the Blazers game in the car and just as I pulled into the parking lot of the hospital, they won the game.

I arrived at about 9PM and immediately was taken for blood work and a chest x-ray. They made sure all the insurance was in place and I was taken to a room at about 11pm. I got a short sleep and was awakened at about 4 am for a blood draw then at 5am I was told that the heart was on the way and I would be "on the table" by 6am. I had been warned throughout the entire process about the possibility of a "dry run" where the doctors may decide that the match is not as good as originally thought but, things seemed to be moving smoothly. It was at this time I learned that sometimes AB positive hearts even are discarded as there is not always a match for them.

I did not know much about my donor except that he was a 44-year-old male with near the same body type as me and disease free. He was someone's father, brother, uncle or son. I could not imagine what that family must be going through but, I was thankful that I would be able to receive such a special gift.

As they rolled me into the operating room and I climbed onto the operating table, I was surprisingly calm. I saw Matthew as they rolled me toward the elevators and told him how proud I was and that I loved him. I had spoken to Casey earlier and let her know the same and that I was so sorry I wouldn't be at her graduation. Being as gracious as she always was, she said that the transplant was so much more important than walking across the stage and that she would be out to see me soon. That was all I needed. I was ready to accept my fate, whatever it was, I realized that I had lived a pretty amazing life and would accept whatever happened next. I would fight as hard as I could to come out on the other side of this surgery but, had truly accepted wherever I was heading next. I was at peace with my family and kind of thought of this as being like I was at the top of a huge rollercoaster. Looking down on the long drop but, knowing there was no way to get off the ride now. It was a strange peace that maybe I had never known. I put my trust in the Higher Power and was completely ready to go.

I remember having a quick visit with Dr. Koomalsingh and joking around with the team prepping me for surgery. I reminded him that I wanted to see photos of the "before and after" hearts and he assured me that would happen. I then remember the anesthesiologist standing over me and asking me if I wanted any music while I was going under. Being the music geek that I am, I started naming off songs. He then told me; the process would only take one song before I was out. I immediately knew what that song would be. Even if it was the last song I ever heard. Then I heard the voice of Roger Waters. "Hello, hello, hello. Is there anybody in there? Just nod if you can hear me. Is there anyone home...There is no pain, you are receding..." As I became "Comfortably Numb" a tear from each eye ran down my face.

CHAPTER EIGHT

"...just the basic facts, can you show me where it hurts. Your lips move but, I can't hear what you say...My hands felt like two balloons, now I've got that feeling once again. I can not explain. This is not how I am..."

I was told by the medical team that I would be in a medically induced coma for 48-72 hours. I started waking up at about 6 am the very next day. My eyes opened slowly, and everything was fuzzy. As my vision started to adjust, I realized that I was alive! I had made it through! I couldn't see much or move my head or neck as the drugs they had given me were still in control but, I could see the clock on the wall said 6:00 and I fully realized where I was and what had been done. Moment later a nurse came into the room and explained why my arms were tied to the bed and that the breathing tube was still in my throat. Matthew had been sleeping in the waiting area and came into the room shortly after the nurse did. Then it was official. I was back! This was REAL! I was living with someone else's heart pumping in my chest. I was still on too much morphine to feel anything yet but, I knew I was alive. Matthew grabbed my tablet a few hours later and I was able to watch my amazing daughter Casey complete a major part of her journey by walking across the stage at George Mason University as a Law School Graduate! Despite my situation, I was so very happy! The pain was not as bad as I had imagined it would be. I had wires coming out of my neck, a few IV's, an external pacemaker still attached and two fluid tubes coming from just below my ribcage. Believe it or not, I was able to manage the pain with only three 5mg morphine tablets the first day and extra strength Tylenol after that. Everyone kept telling me not to be a "tough guy" but, I guess I have a pretty high threshold for pain. Matthew did a great job at keeping the family updated on my status.

The tube finally came out of my throat at about noon. I had almost no voice as there was swelling and possibly light damage done to my vocal cords. I was able to whisper for a short video Matthew sent to his sister at a luncheon after her graduation. I was able to tell her how proud of her I was, that I loved her but, not much else.

As the morphine began to wear off, I realized that my left arm from the shoulder was numb and I could not move it at all. The doctor who came to follow up with me said that the surgery went very well but, sometimes the surgeons "nick a nerve" in patient's chests that runs to another part of the body. He said that this "should heal" but, we would keep an eye on it. As time passed, I began to be able to move the arm. The numbness started subsiding. First to the elbow, then to the wrist. It took a few months before the hand started to heal and nine months later, I still have numbness in my fingers and can not bend my left thumb at the knuckle. One of the small trade offs for having a fully functioning heart. I kept saying, "if that is the worst thing that happens, then I am in pretty awesome shape!" I also woke up looking like "Fat Bastard" in the Austin Powers movies. My hands and feet were so swollen as well as my face. I just wanted to get up and say "Get In my belly"

I started to be able to eat soft foods the next day and they had me drinking many Ensure shakes to add as much protein as possible. Suzie and her Mom showed up the next day to watch the Trailblazers at Denver with me for game seven of that series which the Blazers won to advance to the Western Conference Finals. They had to watch quietly as I was still in ICU. They came to visit the next day and then headed back to Portland. Matthew also had to head back to LA to get back to work. The physical rehab team came in about 28 hours after I woke up and had me on my feet and walking about 150 feet with a high walker. There were tons of wires and tubes still attached but, we got the job done! They came back to visit me every day as I continued to get stronger and I gained the strength to walk farther and farther. At this time, I was attached to five different IV's a day. Some constant, others temporary. And there were 62 pills a day to take initially including the ever important anti-viral and anti-rejection meds that I will be taking for the rest of my life.

I stayed in ICU for a few days then was moved to my own room with a view of Washington Huskies football stadium. I continued to get stronger and walk farther with the help of the physical therapy team. Then I began to walk on my own without the help of a walker. There were struggles every day but, those became farther and farther apart. I was able to leave the hospital after just 17 days and move into the Transplant House, an apartment that is designed for transplant patients who do not live in the area. After transplant there are numerous doctor visits, blood draws and biopsies, to be sure you are not rejecting the new heart and to be sure you continue to improve.

There was one major challenge that no one ever tells you about and that is dealing with insurance. When I went into the hospital, I was completely covered by the Oregon Health Plan and was on Social Security Disability since I died, and the full journey began two years ago. While I was still in Intensive Care and before my voice started to improve, I got a visit from the Social Services team saying that my health coverage would be ending on May 31, 2019. Then I would be switched over to Medicaid automatically as I had been on disability for two years. No warning, just a big surprise that had to be handled Immediately. With virtually no voice I had to start making phone calls to the State of Oregon and to the Social Security department. My social worker also got involved and pointed me in the right direction suggesting that I get supplemental insurance immediately or, I would be responsible for all my meds and for at least twenty percent of the total bill. This would be the first "stress test" of the new heart. I spent hours on the phone with large amounts of that time on hold. Since I was over 50, I qualified for AARP and chose their supplemental insurance plan and their prescription plan. This turned out to be the smartest move I could make. There were also issues about who would be paying the $3,000. per month rent for living in the Transplant House for three and a half months. The manager of the Transplant House, my social worker and Providence Hospital in Portland all got together to be sure I was completely covered. It was a struggle but, I am so glad we found a solution that worked for everyone.

The first of twelve biopsies happened while I was still in the hospital. I was nervous as I knew this would be the biggest test of all to see how good the heart match was and to be sure my body was not rejecting the new heart. During this time there were bi-weekly blood draws to be sure the Tacrolimus and Mycophenolate were working to suppress my immune system. This is important because the body's immune system will attack the foreign object in your chest, the new heart, if it is not suppressed. I was also on heavy doses of Prednisone, which is a steroid that fights infection but, causes damage to your bones and muscles if taken too long. Also, it causes you to have excess swelling and weight, especially the face, belly, hands and legs. The first of the biopsies went perfectly with a zero percent rejection. The doctors kept telling me that I should not worry as just about every patient has some rejection. If it is a small rejection they adjust the Tacrolimus, if it is more serious you may have to spend some time back in the hospital and if it is very serious you get back in the line and wait for another heart.

Not only did the first biopsy have zero-point zero percent rejection but the next nine after that were perfect. Absolutely no rejection. My post-transplant coordinator, Wei continues to tell me what a miracle this is as it almost never happens. This is the biggest proof that the two-year wait was worth the struggle as I have found the perfect match. It is too bad that dating services do not have the same technology to match hearts when people are looking for a soulmate. Imagine how much money they would make then! And, I'm sure the divorce rate would drop dramatically. Initially, Suzie was supposed to spend the first ten days watching over me. I was already moving around very well and even was cooking and doing laundry. She was only able to stay two days as there were many issues at her house in Portland. There were problems with the neighbors, her ex-husband died, and her daughter was having emotional problems. Plus, her mom was about to go through a valve replacement surgery that was supposed to be a simple procedure. As she was trying to find reasons to stay, she got pink eye the second day. As I have no immune system, she had to leave and take care of things at her house so I would not get pink eye. Casey was scheduled to come out to Portland for the remainder of the three months after ten days, as she was taking care of things after graduation to prepare to take the Pennsylvania Bar Exam after she returned from Seattle. I spent the next week alone with no problems, even though I was very careful. Except for March 31st, just three weeks after transplant, when I decided to walk the half mile uphill to a small venue called the Neptune Theatre to see one of my favorite bands. The Record Company was playing, and it was not a sellout. Now, I had been instructed not to be around large crowds yet. Normally, I get there early and stand in the pushing crowd against the stage. I got there early to be sure I got a ticket; I met the band and took photos pre-show and then went up to the balcony to watch the show with virtually no one around me and wearing a mask. It was a great time but, I was completely exhausted the next day.

Casey arrived to babysit me June 1st, and she spent eight or more hours a day studying to take the bar in July. Basically, Casey was there to be sure I took my meds, that I did not try to lift too much or push myself too hard. (Which I have been known to do) She came with me to most of my doctor appointments and biopsies during the time she was there. It was a joy having her there as we traded cooking dinners every other night, did the grocery shopping together and as I got stronger, did many of the tourist things around Seattle like Pikes Place Market, The Mo Pop Museum of Music, a Seattle Mariners game and a few movies. I began walking up and down the hills of Seattle every day and within a month I was up to over five miles a day. I was under what the team called "sternal precautions" which included no driving, no lifting over five pounds, no lifting anything over my head and no running. There were some minor issues along the way but, the medical team was amazed with my fast progress. They called me their "Rock and Roll Transplant Poster Child" on a regular basis. I made my return to radio while I was in the Seattle, taking a part time job recording news for the USA Radio Network. They are an all-news network that ships national news stories to over 400 radio stations and two XM channels around the country. The best part about this gig is that I could do it from home. I had my computer brought to Seattle and as my voice continued to get stronger, my newscasts continued to improve. Casey went back to Pennsylvania on July 17, 2019 and took the Bar Exam on July 30th. She got her passing results a few months later and began working for a law firm in Harrisburg, PA. Her first solo case went to trial in January 2020. She won the case.

Before leaving Seattle, I began having pains as if someone was sticking me with needles inside my chest. I asked Wei what would be causing this. She said, "Oh, I guess we did not tell you but, the nerves to the old heart are severed and not reattached to the new heart. The nerves are waking up now. You should expect this on and off throughout the first two years as each one wakes up." This was not a severe pain; it was just a surprise.

As my recovery was ahead of schedule, I was then cleared to return to Portland

CHAPTER NINE

Labor Day weekend 2019 with a large bucket list of things that I wanted to do. I want to advocate for transplant patients and show that just because you have challenges in your life, you don't give up. You don't sit in the corner saying, "Woe is me". Get up! Live! Be happy and positive! Be as strong as your physical limits allow! At four months after transplant, I was invited to throw a first pitch at a minor league baseball playoff game between the Salem Keizer Volcanoes and the Hillsboro Hops. The announcer talked about the transplant and about helping groups like Donate Life North West as I threw a strike. I did pull a muscle and my shoulder and chest hurt for a few days but, overall it was amazing. I did ten minutes of stand-up comedy at Harvey's Comedy Club in Portland the next day.

I have had a microphone on my hand since age fifteen and that was the scariest thing I had ever done with a mic. I even made jokes about the Heart Transplant process and recovery. I'm not sure If I got sympathy laughs, but the crowd seemed to enjoy my ten-minute set. Then a few weeks later I returned to Coos Bay and jumped on stage and sang six songs with a local band. Then came the biggest physical test of all on September 28th. I had been an athlete in high school and college but, hated long distance running. I decided I would run in a non-competitive 5K Run. It was called the Blacklight Run. It was held at night and they were shooting chalk and paint into the air to run through. I jogged half and ran half but, did not walk and even sprinted the last half mile. I finished in about 40 minutes and was told that put my time in the middle of all the runners. My goal was only to finish and not finish last. Future goals include writing this book, doing more stand up comedy, and advocating as much as possible for all transplant patients.

CHAPTER TEN

Commonly Asked Questions

When you die and are revived or whenever you have a major surgery people always have questions and they are usually not afraid to ask. I have no problem answering them to help educate.

1) Did you see anything while you were dead?

There was no "bright light" and I did not see angels. I think that is an image people think of from the movies. The one thing I do remember was having long versions of dreams that were choppy. Kind of like whenever someone is about to crash a car and says their "life flashed before their eyes". I had all happy dreams of times with my children, watching them grow up, playing sports, cheerleading, winning awards, times in radio interviewing celebrities and local folks and great times with friends and music. Lots of music.

2) Do you feel different with a new heart?

Yes, absolutely! The first thing that I noticed was the feeling like horses   running inside my chest. I also still feel at times like a puppy on a leash, that wants to run in the sunshine and does not want to be harnessed.

3) Do you feel different emotionally?

This is a more complicated question to answer and explain. There is the old saying that "certain people will be in your heart forever". I have noticed that the people who I have stayed in touch with and people who showed they cared during the transplant journey are still a part of my thoughts but, certain people who I cared about have disappeared from "my heart". Not sure if that makes sense but, it is the only way I can explain it. I have always had what people call "deja vous" for very short periods of time. Since my death and revival, and even more after the transplant, I can actually see the place I have never been or the show I have never watched or the person I have never met for a longer period of time and sometimes know what is coming next. I cannot change or control the situation in any but see it happening for a much longer period.

4) Do you look at life differently now?

I am not sure if I look at life differently but, I do things with more passion. I care more about others than ever before. I didn't fear much in life before but, now the only thing I fear is something happening to my children. I have lived eight of my nine lives already and like Rocky, I keep getting up off the mat every time I get knocked down. I have been battered and have the battle scars to prove it. I will never give up and I look at every challenge like I will not be beat.

5) Do you have to take medicine forever?

Yes, there are some medicines I will have to take for the rest of my life. I started at 62 pills a day and am now down to just 19 pills each day. Many of these are supplements but, I will take the anti-rejection pills for the rest of my days.

6) Do you have to change your diet with a transplant?

Yes. I had already started cutting out red meat and sodium before the transplant. Now I have the added challenge of eliminating anything that may cause any food born illness as my body does not have the ability to fight it. What may be a small stomach for someone else could become food poisoning for a transplant patient. I am now not able to eat my favorite food, Sushi. I cook all red meat, pork, fish or poultry well done. Why would you bother having a prime rib, for example, if you couldn't have it medium-rare? Processed lunchmeats are not allowed unless cooked to get any potential bacteria out of it. Veggies need to be washed numerous times if raw but, it is suggested that they all be cooked for at least the first two years. No food from buffets, or family picnics as they may have been out too long. No ice or sodas from fountain machines as you have no idea how clean they are kept. Stay away from fast food and only go to restaurants that have high cleanliness ratings. I don't bother with sodium as I lost my taste for salt by not having any for two years. No canned veggies, only fresh ones.

I have had to reintroduce different foods into my diet. Just like being a baby all over again. Some foods work and others do not. And others I can eat but, fully understand that I will be taking extra Tums afterward.

CHAPTER ELEVEN

What Comes Next?

I have moved into my own place, set up my recording studio and continue working for the news network. I have begun to look more long term toward the future and am have been cleared to participate in the 2020 Transplant Games in the Meadowlands, New Jersey, July 2020. I hope to participate in basketball, a few track and field events and the fun Lyrics for Life competition. This event is just like the Olympics but, limited to transplant patients and donors only.

I learned that the world record for living after a Heart Transplant was 33 years. That record continues to grow as the person who has it, is still alive. I hope to break that record one day. I have so much to live for. Plus, it may be many years before I get to see grandchildren. No need to rush, Matthew and Casey. Take your time and enjoy your lives!

Two months after my transplant I sent a five-page letter to the donor family through the agency that handles connecting donor families with the transplant recipients. I am hoping to get a response as I would like to show my extreme gratitude personally to the family and show them that his heart is being put to good use. I understand that their grief may initially be too hard to handle, but I do hope they find the strength to meet someday. Much like adoption of children, the donor family does have the right to stay anonymous.

I think the reason that I was drawn to the west coast, though I did not understand it at first, was to force me to slow down my insane pace. Since I have been here, I now know that doing the work is important, but allowing things to happen can be just as precious.

I have learned that hard work brings results but, overwork can kill you. Take the time to enjoy life. Do not let your stress or the stress of the people around you bring you down. If their stress is to much for you to handle, whenever possible separate yourself from it. Be happy. Love your life and the people you allow to be in your inner circle.

Sting said "Nothing comes from violence. Nothing ever could. For all us born beneath an angry star. Lest we forget how fragile we are. "

I thank everyone who was as part of this journey with me. Whether you were standing next to me, rooting for me from afar or just liked a random Facebook update. I appreciate all of you. The ones I know now and those will stand beside me in the future. Remember, the Beatles said, "All You Need Is Love"

And yes, The Heart of Rock and Roll Is Still Beating...In Portland. Thanks Huey.

www.ingramcontent.com/pod-product-compliance
Lightning Source LLC
Chambersburg PA
CBHW030534220526
45463CB00007B/2835